SHARON LUCIE TAYLOR

Easy Exercises for Strong Glutes

Learn to Power your Motion with the Largest and Most Powerful Muscles in Your Body

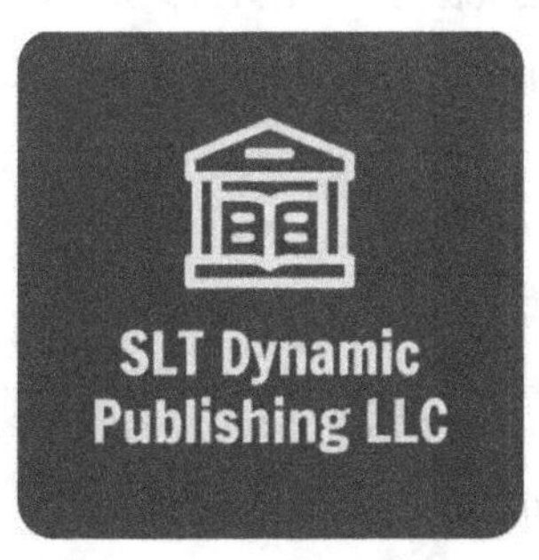

Contents

Introduction   1

1   Chapter 1   5

What Are the Glute Muscles and the Benefits of
Strengthening Them?   5

2   Chapter 2   10

How Can We Describe All of the Exercises in This
Book as Easy?   10

    Adaptability to All Levels   11

    Little to No Equipment Needed   12

    Controlled, Slow Movements   12

    Low-Impact with High Engagement   13

    Exercises Adapt to Your Progress   13

3   Chapter 3   15

Isolating the Glutes   15

    Why Isolate the Glutes?   16

    Techniques for Isolating the Glutes   16

      Progressive Glute Contraction   17

      Mind-Muscle Connection   17

      Proper Form and Range of Motion   18

      Progressive Overload   18

      Hip Thrusts   19

      Glute Bridges   19

      Cable Kickbacks and Variations   20

      Clamshells with Resistance Band   22

      Bulgarian Split Squats   23

Step-Ups with Hip Extension 23

4 Chapter 4 25

Mind-Muscle Connection 25

Techniques for Strengthening the Mind-Muscle Connection 26

Pre-Activation Warm-Up 26

Slow Down Each Rep 26

Pause at the Peak Contraction 27

Adjust Foot Placement and Positioning 27

Use Resistance Bands for Extra Tension 28

Visualize the Muscle Working 28

Lighten the Load to Focus on Form 28

Push Through the Heels 29

Contract at the Start of Each Movement 29

Practice Static Holds and Isometric Contractions 30

Putting It All Together: Building Your Mind-Muscle Connection 30

5 Chapter 5 31

Proper Form and Range of Motion 31

Critical Techniques for Proper Form and Range of Motion 32

Maintain a Neutral Spine 32

Focus on Hip-Hinging 32

Keep Your Knees Aligned with Your Toes 32

Limit Knee Bend in Certain Movements 33

Use a Controlled, Full Range of Motion 33

Engage Your Core Throughout the Movement 34

Keep Your Feet Positioned Correctly 34

Avoid Excessive Leaning or Tilting 34

Monitor Your Pelvic Position in Glute Bridges and Hip Thrusts 36

Gradually Increase Weight to Maintain Control 36

Putting Proper Form into Practice   36

6   Chapter 6   38

Progressive Overload   38

Ways to Implement Progressive Overload   39

Gradually Increase Weight or Resistance   39

Add Resistance Bands   39

Increase Reps or Sets   40

Slow Down the Tempo   40

Increase Range of Motion (ROM)   40

Use Single-Leg Variations for Added Challenge   41

Increase the Frequency of Glute Workouts   41

Incorporate Heavier Compound Lifts   42

Reduce Rest Time Between Sets   42

Experiment with Drop Sets   42

Applying Progressive Overload Consistently   43

7   Chapter 7   44

Glute Strength in Everyday Activities   44

Tips for Activating Your Glutes in Everyday Activities   45

Bending and Lifting   45

Walking   45

Stair Climbing   46

Standing Up from a Chair   48

Maintaining Proper Posture Throughout the Day   49

8   Chapter 8   51

Using Glutes in Combination Exercises   51

Lunges with Overhead Press   51

Deadlifts with Row   53

Squat to Shoulder Press   55

Step-Up to Knee Raise   55

Bulgarian Split Squat with Bicep Curl   55

Making Glute Activation a Habit   56

9 Conclusion   57
   References   60

Introduction

Why Strong Glutes Matter

Have you ever struggled with daily activities that used to be easy? Maybe you've noticed that lifting things, climbing stairs, or even just walking has become more challenging. That's exactly how I felt when I decided to write this book. I'd always enjoyed going for walks, but I reached a point where those walks no longer felt invigorating—they felt like the only exercise I could manage. I had become what I like to call a "deconditioned" person, someone whose body had lost strength and resilience over time. Everyday tasks became less easy, and I could feel myself over-stressing my back because my arms and legs were not as strong as they used to be (Biel, 2014).

When I first tried to improve my overall strength by working out, I assumed the solution was simply strengthening my legs. However, focusing on exercises for my quadriceps (the muscles in the front of my thighs) and the back of my legs only led to knee pain. It didn't take long for me to realize I was missing something. After researching exercise and its effects on knee health, I discovered that one of the main culprits for my knee pain was how I walked and used my muscles during exercise and daily movement. I relied too much on my quadriceps muscles (called quads) and not enough on another major muscle group: my glutes (McGill, 2015; Weak Glutes Are Affecting Your Knee Pain!, 2024).

Through research, I learned that the glute muscles—the gluteus maximus, gluteus medius, and gluteus minimus—are the largest and most powerful muscles in the body. They are crucial in stabilizing the hips, supporting the spine, and creating efficient movement (DeLuca, 2015). When adequately engaged, they can reduce the strain on other muscles, including the quads, hamstrings, and lower back. For many of us, however, these muscles remain underutilized, forcing other, smaller muscles to compensate. This compensation makes movement inefficient and increases the risk of injuries, such as knee and lower back pain (Contreras & Schoenfeld, 2011).

I was fascinated by this information and excited to put it into practice. I started experimenting with exercises and techniques that shifted the work from my quads to my glutes. The results were remarkable: my knee pain decreased, I could walk longer distances without discomfort, and daily activities started to feel easier. With stronger glutes, I felt more balanced, stable, and capable (McGill, 2015).

Why I Wrote This Book

This journey of self-discovery led me to write this book because I knew I couldn't be the only one facing these challenges. I realized that many people, regardless of age or fitness level, could benefit from stronger glutes. Whether it's due to sedentary lifestyles, repetitive movements, or simply the effects of aging, many of us risk losing strength in our glutes without even realizing it. However, with some targeted effort, we can regain that strength and experience authentic, tangible benefits in our daily lives (Biel, 2014).

This book aims to help readers like you build a stronger foundation through glute-focused workouts. Strong glutes can make everyday tasks easier, relieve knee and lower back stress, and allow more efficient, powerful movement. Strengthening the glutes also improves posture, balance, and overall physical resilience (Contreras & Schoenfeld, 2011).

What This Book Covers

In this book, we'll dive into everything you need to know about glute strength: why it's important, how to engage the muscles properly, and which exercises are most effective. We begin by exploring the anatomy and function of the glutes, examining what these muscles are, how they work, and why they're essential for daily movement. Understanding the role of the glutes and how they interact with other muscle groups provides a clearer picture of how your body moves and highlights potential areas where imbalances may arise (DeLuca, 2015).

Next, we address the role of glute strength in relieving pain and preventing injury. Strong glutes protect your knees, lower back, and ankles by effectively absorbing and distributing movement forces. This section also covers common causes of knee and back pain associated with weak glutes. It explains how targeted strengthening can help alleviate these issues (McGill, 2015).

We then move on to practical techniques for activating the glutes. Learning to "wake up" and engage the glutes is foundational in building strength, particularly for those with underactive glutes due to prolonged sitting. This section offers tips for activating your glutes in workouts and everyday life (Contreras & Schoenfeld, 2011).

The book includes a curated selection of glute exercises that are simple, effective, and require minimal equipment. Starting with foundational movements like glute bridges and hip thrusts, we progress to more advanced exercises, such as single-leg variations and resistance band exercises, that further target and strengthen the glutes (Biel, 2014).

To maintain progress, we cover progressive overload and long-term strength building. Consistent results require progressively challenging the muscles, so this section provides guidance on safely increasing resistance and intensity to keep the glutes growing stronger without overloading the joints (DeLuca, 2015).

Finally, we explore ways to incorporate glute strength into everyday activities. Strong glutes improve movement beyond the gym, and we discuss how to apply your newfound strength in daily tasks, from lifting to climbing stairs, making your routine more efficient and physically supported (McGill, 2015).

Important Precautions

Before you start an exercise program, consultation with a healthcare practitioner is highly recommended. This is especially important if you have pre-existing health conditions or concerns. This book provides general information on exercise techniques and does not substitute for personalized medical advice. Please consult your healthcare professional to assess your health needs and help ensure that an exercise plan is safe and suitable. Please prioritize your health and safety by seeking professional guidance when needed (OpenAI, 2024).

1

Chapter 1

What Are the Glute Muscles and the Benefits of Strengthening Them?

While the glutes are often associated with shaping our backsides, their role extends far beyond aesthetics. As the body's largest and most powerful muscle group, the glutes are the driving force behind our everyday movements, balance, and stability. They support nearly everything we do, from standing to running to lifting, making them essential for our everyday function and long-term physical health. In this chapter, you'll learn about the glute muscles—their structure, functions, and importance—and understand why strengthening them can impact how you move and feel.

The glutes, technically called the gluteal muscles, are made up of three primary muscles located in the back of the hip and thigh region. Working together, these muscles help stabilize the pelvis, support posture, and generate the power needed for lower-body activities like walking, running, and jumping (McGill, 2015).

The gluteus maximus, the largest and most visible of these glute muscles, is a powerhouse in maintaining posture and stabilizing the pelvis during movement. Its primary functions include extending the hip, rotating it outward, and moving the leg away from the body. The gluteus maximus is an essential player in exercises such as hip thrusts, squats, and deadlifts, where its power and size make it a significant source of strength (Collins, 2019; Naskar, 2023).

The gluteus medius, the next glute muscle in line, is a key player in preventing hip and knee injuries. It is responsible for hip abduction, the action of moving the leg outward, and for stabilizing the pelvis during movements like walking or balancing on one leg. It also assists in rotating the thigh, helping you turn your legs inward or outward. When you perform exercises such as lateral band walks, clamshells, or side-lying hip abductions, the gluteus medius is hard at work, ensuring your lower-body stability. (McGill, 2015)

The gluteus minimus is the smallest of the three glute muscles and is located beneath the gluteus medius. Though small, it works closely with the gluteus medius to assist in hip abduction and helps to stabilize the pelvis during movement. It also aids in thigh rotation, supporting various motions that involve turning the leg (McGill, 2015). While exercises don't often specifically target the gluteus minimus, movements that work the gluteus medius, like side lunges and clamshells, also engage this muscle, supporting hip function and providing the necessary balance and stability for smooth, controlled movement (Contreras & Schoenfeld, 2011; Richter, 2023).

Strong glutes aren't just for athletes or fitness enthusiasts; they provide benefits that enhance everyday life. Glute strength is foundational for many athletic movements, creating the power needed for fast, explosive actions such as running, jumping, and sprinting. With strong glutes, athletes can increase their speed, agility, and overall performance (DeLuca, 2015). However, glute strength also plays a critical role in maintaining good posture and stability for everyone, not just athletes. The glutes support the pelvis and spine alignment, helping us stand upright and reducing strain on the lower back. They keep the pelvis stable during activities like walking or single-leg exercises, making it easier to move with balance and precision. This means that strong glutes can make everyday tasks feel easier and less tiring, empowering you to move with confidence and comfort (McGill, 2015).

When the glutes are weak, other muscles, such as the quads and lower back, are forced to do more work than they are meant to handle. This often results in compensations that can lead to injury over time. Strong glutes, by contrast, absorb the impact forces involved in movement, protecting the knees, lower back, and hamstrings from overuse. With well-developed glutes, daily tasks like lifting, bending, and climbing stairs become easier and less tiring, as these muscles provide the foundation for stability and strength in lower-body motions. This reduces the likelihood of strains or falls and makes day-to-day tasks feel less taxing. By strengthening your glutes, you're not just improving your physical health, you're also creating a protective shield against potential injuries, giving you a sense of security and confidence in your movements (McGill, 2015).

In addition to stability, strong glutes offer core and pelvic support. They relieve pressure from the spine, particularly for those who experience lower back pain or have weak pelvic muscles. Glute strength encourages better core engagement by reinforcing the connection between the pelvis and lower spine, creating a more stable foundation for the entire body (DeLuca, 2015). Beyond the physical ease and support, training the glutes also benefits metabolism. Because they are the largest muscle group in the body, strengthening them increases overall muscle mass, which boosts the resting metabolic rate. This increase aids in weight management and calorie burn, even when you're not exercising, making glute strength beneficial for fitness and health (Contreras & Schoenfeld, 2011).

Weak glutes can cause a chain reaction of muscular imbalances throughout the body, reducing movement efficiency and increasing injury risk. When the glutes aren't functioning at their best, smaller muscles, like the hamstrings, quads, and lower back muscles, have to compensate for what the glute muscles are not doing. This compensation strains these muscles and often leads to overuse injuries or chronic discomfort. Over time, these imbalances can create knee pain, hip discomfort, or even lower back issues, turning simple, everyday movements into sources of pain and difficulty. However, there's hope. Strengthening the glutes helps correct these imbalances, encouraging efficient and pain-free movement patterns. By focusing on glute strengthening, you can not only prevent these issues but also correct existing imbalances, giving you a sense of optimism and control over your physical health (Biel, 2014; Collins, 2019).

This book will equip you with practical and effective exercises that engage all three glute muscles. It will help you build glute strength in a balanced way that supports all aspects of your physical health. The exercises are straightforward and adaptable, allowing you to start from any fitness level and progress at your own pace. Each chapter will introduce new techniques and specific guidance on activating, isolating, and strengthening the glutes safely and effectively (DeLuca, 2015).

As you move through the book, you'll gain a strong understanding of the glutes' essential role in your movement and stability and be equipped with a powerful toolkit for creating long-lasting physical resilience. By strengthening these muscles, you're not just supporting your fitness—you're investing in a healthier, more active lifestyle. This chapter lays the foundation for a journey toward stronger glutes and a stronger, more capable you. The following chapters will delve into specific exercises, proper form, and progressive techniques to ensure that each workout you do maximizes your glutes' strength, stability, and function (Contreras & Schoenfeld, 2011).

$$2$$

Chapter 2

How Can We Describe All of the Exercises in This Book as Easy?

We can describe these exercises as "easy" because they are adaptable, require minimal equipment, and focus on simple, controlled movements that allow you to gradually build strength. They do not require advanced skills or fitness levels needed to do complex exercises or high-impact exercises, so these movements are accessible to beginners and provide effective results without overloading the body (Biel, 2014). Here's how each characteristic supports the ease of these exercises:

Adaptability to All Levels

These exercises are not just for beginners or advanced exercisers but for everyone. They can be tailored to match each person's fitness level, making them accessible and practical. For beginners, starting with bodyweight versions is ideal, as it allows them to focus on mastering form and building a solid foundation without the added stress of extra weight. Exercises like glute bridges, clamshells, and lunges can be done without weights to ensure proper technique and muscle engagement (Contreras & Schoenfeld, 2011). Beginners may also use lighter resistance bands, providing enough tension to activate the glutes without overwhelming other muscle groups. This approach ensures manageable movements and allows beginners to develop a solid mind-muscle connection.

For those with more experience, increasing the weight or resistance adds a greater challenge, allowing them to build strength progressively. Advanced exercisers can add weights, such as dumbbells or barbells, to exercises like hip thrusts, squats, and step-ups, which enhances the intensity and targets the glutes more deeply. They can also use heavier resistance bands around the thighs for exercises like lateral band walks or hip abductions, providing additional tension that further activates the gluteus medius and minimus. Advanced exercisers might also incorporate single-leg variations, such as single-leg hip thrusts or single-leg deadlifts, to isolate each glute independently, increasing the intensity and balance required for each movement (DeLuca, 2015). This flexibility in approach empowers everyone to start at a level right for them and progress gradually as they build strength and confidence. People of all abilities can adjust these movements by modifying weight, resistance, and exercise variations.

Little to No Equipment Needed

Many exercises in this book are designed to be effective using either no or minimal equipment, making them suitable for at-home workouts or spaces without access to a full gym. For example, glute bridges are a powerful bodyweight exercise that targets the gluteus maximus and can be done on any flat surface, making them ideal for beginners and easy to perform anywhere. Variations like single-leg glute bridges add intensity without needing weights, increasing the engagement on each side for a more challenging workout (McGill, 2015).

Clamshells are another bodyweight option that targets the gluteus medius and minimus, aiding in hip stability and pelvic alignment. This exercise requires only a mat and, for an added challenge, a resistance band placed above the knees. Clamshells are especially valuable for isolating the glutes in a controlled, low-impact way. They are easily incorporated into a warm-up or main workout routine (Biel, 2014).

Controlled, Slow Movements

Each exercise encourages a slow, controlled pace, emphasizing form and building a solid mind-muscle connection. This approach minimizes impact on the joints by focusing on deliberate, precise movements, reducing unnecessary strain and wear over time (DeLuca, 2015). High-impact exercises, especially when done without proper control, can place undue stress on areas like the knees, hips, and lower back. A slower pace allows you to focus on activating the glutes fully, which supports the surrounding joints and creates a protective effect, helping to prevent injuries associated with poor form or rushed movements. With controlled exercises, the glutes bear the brunt of the work, allowing the joints to move naturally without excess force, making the entire workout safer and easier on the body (Contreras & Schoenfeld, 2011).

This focus on control also supports steady improvement, enabling you to progress gradually without the risk of injury that comes with overloading or performing exercises too quickly. For example, by slowing down movements like hip thrusts, you have time to ensure your glutes engage correctly, allowing each muscle fiber to contribute to the lift (McGill, 2015).

Low-Impact with High Engagement

These exercises focus on isolated muscle engagement, meaning they target one specific muscle group—your glutes—instead of relying on multiple muscles or complex movements. Unlike high-impact or multi-directional exercises that can stress various body parts, isolation exercises are simpler, allowing you to concentrate fully on activating and strengthening your glutes (DeLuca, 2015).

Exercises Adapt to Your Progress

This book is designed with exercises that can grow with the reader, making it adaptable for beginners and advanced exercisers. Each movement in this book has a foundation that's accessible for those just starting out while also offering options to increase intensity and complexity as strength improves. By building a progressive approach, readers can follow along comfortably at their current level and gradually adjust to make exercises more challenging over time. This flexibility ensures that every exercise can meet the needs of beginners while still providing the opportunity for advanced readers to deepen their training (Contreras & Schoenfeld, 2011).

This adaptable approach allows readers to continuously progress, regardless of where they're starting. Beginners can move at their own pace, while advanced exercisers have ample options to push their limits. By following a structured yet flexible program, readers at any level can feel empowered to achieve their goals, knowing they can modify each exercise to keep their glutes growing stronger every step of the way (Biel, 2014).

3

Chapter 3

Isolating the Glutes

For years, I barely used my glutes compared to the other muscles in my body. Whether walking, lifting, or even running, my legs, back, and core did most of the work. My glutes? Almost nothing. The result was that I felt strangely disconnected from these powerful muscles. I realized that it would become easier to walk and do everyday activities if I could find a way to isolate my glutes—focusing on exercises that minimized the involvement of other muscle groups like my quads, hamstrings, and lower back (Biel, 2014). In this chapter, we'll examine what it means to isolate the glutes and why it's beneficial. We will also go through some straightforward exercises to help you do that.

Why Isolate the Glutes?

When we say "isolate the glutes," we're talking about exercises that specifically target and engage the glutes while minimizing the work done by surrounding muscles. This approach helps you concentrate on building a robust mind-muscle connection with your glutes, making it easier to feel them working and ensuring they're truly doing the job. Over time, this focus will help you activate the glutes more naturally in exercise and everyday movements, strengthening them to prevent injury, improve stability, and enhance physical resilience (DeLuca, 2015). The benefits of isolating your glutes are immense, and the journey to a stronger, more resilient body starts here. Imagine the potential improvements in your physical performance, the increased stability, and the reduced risk of injury. Further, mastering these glute isolation exercises will not only build your strength but also fill you with a sense of pride and motivation. Each exercise, whether done with or without added weights, is a testament to your dedication and progress in your fitness journey. (McGill, 2015).

Techniques for Isolating the Glutes

Empower yourself with the knowledge of how to isolate the glutes effectively. By understanding and applying the three main techniques-developing a solid mind-muscle connection, using proper form and range of motion, and implementing progressive overload-you can confidently and safely isolate your glutes.

Progressive Glute Contraction

To enhance your glute tightening, start by sitting with your knees slightly apart. Lightly engage your glutes, contracting them at about 10% of your maximum, and hold for ten seconds. Closing your eyes during this exercise is helpful, as it helps you focus on engaging the glutes only and not any other leg muscles, such as quads. This ten-second hold is crucial as it helps wake up dormant muscle cells by reinforcing the neurological connection between the brain and the glute muscles. To progress, increase the contraction in increments of 5% or 10% of your maximum, continuing for ten seconds each time (*Better Active Your Glutes by Doing THIS*, 2024).

Mind-Muscle Connection

Establishing a solid mind-muscle connection is crucial to isolating and strengthening your glutes. This simple yet powerful technique means actively focusing on contracting the glute muscles during each movement. When you concentrate on feeling the glutes working, you can maximize their engagement and make each repetition more effective. This technique may seem simple, but it's a powerful way to improve your body's connection with the glutes, making every exercise more intentional (Contreras & Schoenfeld, 2011). You can do this, and you will see results. It's a straightforward technique that anyone can apply, and it will make a significant difference in your glute isolation journey.

Proper Form and Range of Motion

When isolating the glutes, it's essential to use the correct form and control your range of motion to avoid over-relying on other muscles like the quads or lower back. Controlled movements keep your glutes as the primary muscles doing the work, ensuring they're fully engaged. This means watching your alignment, keeping the movements slow, and paying attention to your body's cues. Adjust your form or positioning if you feel other muscles taking over (McGill, 2015). Understanding and applying these techniques will give you the confidence and knowledge to isolate your glutes effectively and safely.

Progressive Overload

To continue strengthening the glutes over time, you'll want to implement progressive overload, which means lifting heavier weights and/or increasing resistance as you get stronger. This continual challenge forces the glutes to adapt and grow, ensuring they stay engaged and active. Begin each exercise with lighter weights or resistance bands, then gradually add weight or increase the band resistance as you progress. This approach ensures that your glutes are consistently challenged without overloading other muscles (DeLuca, 2015).

Hip Thrusts

Hip thrusts are ideal for isolating the glutes, especially the gluteus maximus. Sit on the ground with your upper back against a bench to perform a hip thrust. Place your feet flat on the floor and bend your knees. If you don't have a barbell, you can use a heavy object like a backpack filled with books. Lift your hips as you press through your heels until your abdomen and upper legs are parallel to the ground. Focus on squeezing your glutes at the top of the movement, ensuring they're fully engaged, and avoid overarching your back. If you feel your quads taking over, adjust your foot placement slightly farther away from your body (Contreras & Schoenfeld, 2011; Rush, 2024).

Glute Bridges

Glute bridges are similar to hip thrusts but can be done without a bench, making them an accessible option for glute isolation. Lie on your back. Then, put your feet flat on the floor, bending your knees. Rest your arms at your side. Lift your hips by pushing through your heels. Then, squeeze your glutes at the top of the movement. For added resistance, place a band around your thighs. You can also make this exercise more intense by lifting one leg at a time after raising your hips for single-leg bridges, which puts extra focus on each glute (Biel, 2014; Personal Training | Perpetual Movement Fitness | JP Purkey | Boulder, CO, n.d.).

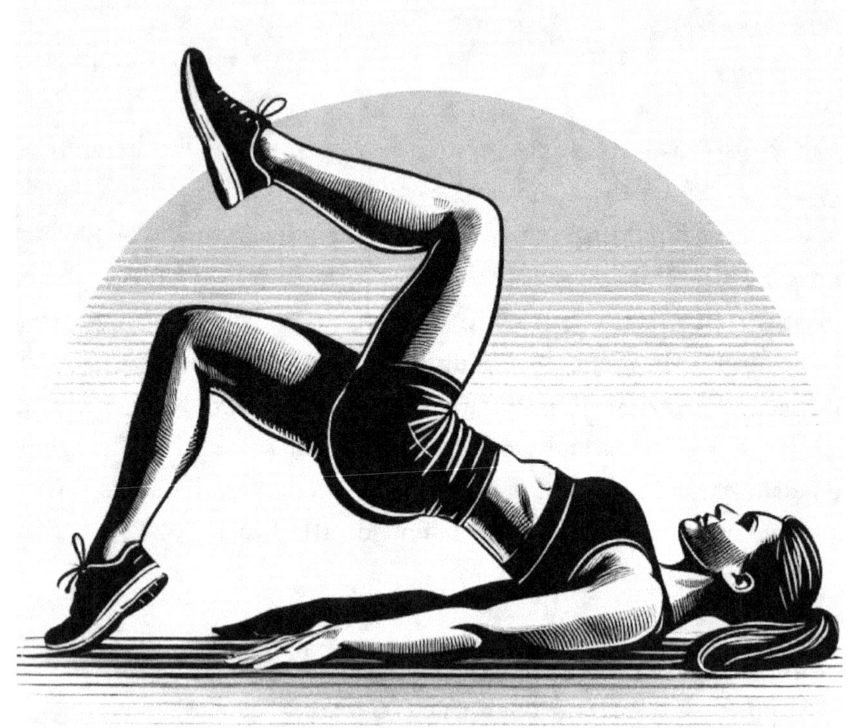

Glute Bridge with Leg Raise

Cable Kickbacks and Variations

Cable kickbacks and variations provide an excellent way to isolate the glutes, specifically the gluteus maximus. These exercises can be done at home or in a gym. There are many variations on the kickback. The easiest versions can be done with no weights or resistance bands. Standing versions involve standing on one leg with the knee slightly bent, lifting the other leg behind you. Floor versions involve lifting one leg behind you while the other knee and both hands support you on the floor. Resistance bands can be used to increase the load on the glutes for either standing or floor kickbacks. The resistance band can be around the ankles, calves, or thighs. Cable kickbacks involve a standing kickback that increases the load on the glutes by attaching weights via a cable and ankle band to the leg that is kicking back.

To perform a cable kickback: Stand on one leg with your knee bent slightly, then extend the leg with the ankle band attached to the cable back in a controlled motion, concentrating on squeezing the glute as you lift. For beginners, it's important to start with a lighter weight and focus on the form. Keep your back straight, core engaged, and avoid any swinging or back involvement to keep the focus on the glutes. Keep the motion slow and controlled, avoiding any swinging or back involvement to keep the focus on the glutes.

Throughout the cable kickback movement, it's important to keep your core engaged and your back straight. This support from your core and back ensures that the focus remains on the glutes, helping you to perform the exercise with confidence and precision. Finally, if you have balance issues, be sure to hold onto a sturdy immovable object while you are performing standing kickbacks. (Coach 2022; McGill, 2015; Rachelle, 2024).

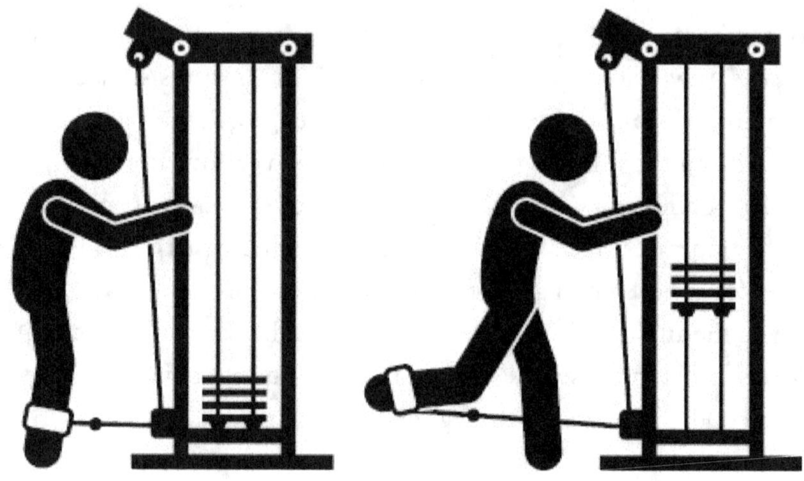

Cable Kickback

Clamshells with Resistance Band

Clamshells are perfect for isolating the gluteus medius and minimus, which help stabilize the hips. To do a clamshell, lie on your side and bend both legs at a 45-degree angle. Open your top leg, keeping your feet together and your hips stable, then slowly lower it back. This movement targets the side glutes, aiding in hip stability and balance. You can exercise with a resistance band above your knees for greater exertion (DeLuca, 2015).

Bulgarian Split Squats

Bulgarian split squats can be an effective exercise for targeting the glutes if you can isolate your glutes while doing this exercise. It can also improve balance and stability, but if you have balance issues, hold onto a stable object nearby, such as a table, refrigerator, wall, etc., so you don't fall over. The important thing is to isolate your glutes, which may be easier if you go slowly and do not bend your standing knee too far (Contreras & Schoenfeld, 2011). Standing a few feet in front of a bench, place one foot on the bench behind you and lower down into a squat on your standing leg. Lean forward slightly to shift the focus to your glutes and drive up through the heel of your front foot.

Step-Ups with Hip Extension

Step-ups provide an effective way to work the glutes without overloading the quads. Standing before a box, bench, or step, place one foot on the surface and squeeze your glutes as you push through your heel to step up. At the top, focus on extending your hip and squeezing your glutes before stepping down. For added resistance, hold dumbbells, focusing on the glutes to lift rather than relying on momentum or pushing off with your trailing leg (Biel, 2014).

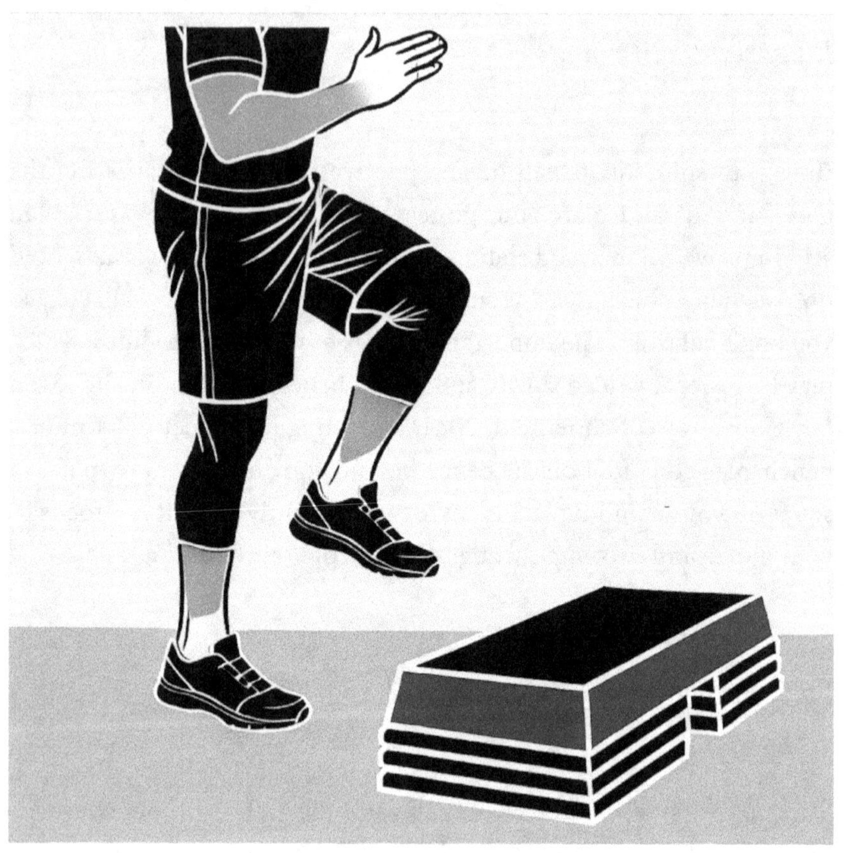

Step-Up

4

Chapter 4

Mind-Muscle Connection

Imagine exercising your glutes and knowing, without a doubt, that each movement is engaging precisely the muscles you want to strengthen. This ability to feel and control your glute muscles is known as the mind-muscle connection. It's a powerful tool for making every rep count, enhancing the effectiveness of your workouts, and bringing intention to each movement (DeLuca, 2015). This chapter will focus on practical ways to build a solid mind-muscle connection with your glutes, helping you isolate and engage them fully while you exercise.

The mind-muscle connection isn't just about physical movement; it's about training your brain to communicate directly with your glutes. Many people experience weak glute activation because they aren't used to intentionally engaging these muscles. By consciously focusing on your glutes, you'll learn to isolate and feel them working, which makes your workouts more efficient and impactful (Contreras & Schoenfeld, 2011). Let's dive into practical techniques to help you deepen this connection and maximize your glute-focused training.

Techniques for Strengthening the Mind-Muscle Connection

Pre-Activation Warm-Up

Starting each workout with a glute-specific warm-up is an excellent way to "wake up" your glutes and prime them for the main exercises. Targeted warm-ups like glute bridges, banded clamshells, or side-lying hip abductions can stimulate your glutes, ensuring they're ready to engage fully. Think of these exercises as a signal to your brain and body that it's time for the glutes to work. This activation technique builds awareness, setting the stage for effective glute engagement during the central part of your workout (Biel, 2014).

Slow Down Each Rep

Rushing through exercises can lead to sloppy form and diminished muscle engagement. When focusing on your glutes, try slowing down each rep, especially during the eccentric phase or the lowering part of the movement. This technique, known as "time under tension," allows you to concentrate on how your glutes feel as they contract and lengthen. Slowing down gives you more control, helping you feel each muscle fiber working (McGill, 2015).

Pause at the Peak Contraction

In exercises like hip thrusts, bridges, or squats, pausing at the movement's peak for a few seconds can make a big difference. At the top, focus on squeezing your glutes as tightly as possible. This pause forces you to fully engage the muscles, increasing awareness and strengthening the connection between your mind and glutes. Over time, this habit will improve your ability to feel the glutes working at every phase of an exercise (Contreras & Schoenfeld, 2011).

Adjust Foot Placement and Positioning

The angle of your feet can influence which muscles engage during an exercise. In movements like squats and lunges, experiment with foot placement. For example, turning your feet slightly outward or placing them a bit wider than usual can help activate different parts of the glutes and reduce quad involvement. Making minor adjustments allows you to feel other areas of the glutes working, giving you more control and ensuring that the glutes, not the surrounding muscles, are the leading players in each exercise (Biel, 2014).

Use Resistance Bands for Extra Tension

Adding a resistance band above your knees during squats, hip thrusts, or side steps can significantly increase glute engagement. The band creates added tension, challenging the glutes throughout the movement, especially in the upward phase. By constantly pushing against the band, you'll notice greater activation in your glutes, reinforcing the mind-muscle connection (DeLuca, 2015).

Visualize the Muscle Working

Visualization is a powerful mental tool for enhancing muscle activation. As you perform each rep, imagine your glutes contracting and relaxing, focusing on the specific movement happening in the muscle. This mental practice can help you concentrate on the target muscle, making it easier to feel and control. Visualizing the action as you perform it bridges the gap between mind and muscle, leading to a more intentional and connected workout (McGill, 2015).

Lighten the Load to Focus on Form

Using lighter weights, especially when just starting, can make establishing a robust mind-muscle connection easier. When the load is too heavy, other muscles may take over, preventing you from fully feeling the glutes at work. By lowering the weight, you can focus more on form and intentionally engaging the glutes, building a solid foundation before progressing to heavier weights (Contreras & Schoenfeld, 2011; Derek).

Push Through the Heels

Paying attention to foot placement, explicitly focusing on pushing through your heels, helps shift the emphasis from the quads to the glutes. In movements like squats, lunges, or hip thrusts, drive through your heels rather than your toes to direct the force to your glutes. This simple adjustment makes a noticeable difference in how the glutes engage, ensuring they take on most of the workload (DeLuca, 2015).

Contract at the Start of Each Movement

One effective cue for engaging your glutes right from the start is to squeeze them slightly before each rep. By contracting the glutes at the beginning of a movement, you ensure they're actively involved from the outset rather than just at the end. This cue can be especially helpful in squats or lunges, where other muscles often want to take over. Starting each rep with a glute contraction sets the tone for the entire movement (Biel, 2014).

Practice Static Holds and Isometric Contractions

Static holds, like standing glute squeezes or wall sits, are valuable tools for building a mind-muscle connection. By holding a contraction, you can feel the glutes working without the distraction of movement. Practicing static holds helps you isolate and feel the glute contraction more distinctly, reinforcing the mental focus on your glutes (McGill, 2015).

Putting It All Together: Building Your Mind-Muscle Connection

Establishing a solid mind-muscle connection with your glutes can make each workout more effective and help you get the most out of every exercise. By integrating these techniques, you'll gain greater control over your movements, ensuring that the glutes are the primary muscles doing the work. Mindful glute engagement may take time to develop. Still, as you practice, you'll notice your glutes responding more naturally and consistently (Contreras & Schoenfeld, 2011; Pt, 2023).

A powerful mind-muscle connection will enhance your physical awareness, making your exercises more impactful and safer, as you'll be less likely to rely on other muscle groups that aren't meant to bear the brunt of the movement. As you progress with your glute training, remember that the quality of each rep matters more than quantity. By training your mind to connect with your glutes, you'll unlock the full potential of these powerful muscles, helping you move with confidence, control, and strength (DeLuca, 2015).

5

Chapter 5

Proper Form and Range of Motion

Building strong, resilient glutes isn't just about lifting heavy weights or doing endless repetitions. One of the most critical aspects of glute training is using proper form and a controlled range of motion. This focus ensures that you're targeting the glutes effectively while minimizing strain on surrounding muscles like the quads or lower back. Without the proper form, other muscle groups may take over, reducing the effectiveness of your workout and potentially leading to injury (McGill, 2015). This chapter provides essential guidelines for using the correct form and range of motion to keep your movements safe, controlled, and glute-focused.

Critical Techniques for Proper Form and Range of Motion

Maintain a Neutral Spine

One of the most important form basics is to maintain a neutral spine. This means keeping your back flat and avoiding any arching or rounding. Exercises like hip thrusts, squats, and deadlifts place significant stress on the lower back, so it's essential to stabilize your spine by engaging your core. Imagine tucking your pelvis slightly to maintain a neutral position; this adjustment reduces strain on the lower back, allowing you to focus on activating the glutes (Contreras & Schoenfeld, 2011).

Focus on Hip-Hinging

Hip-hinging is critical to isolating the glutes while minimizing quad engagement in exercises like deadlifts or Romanian deadlifts. Instead of bending at the knees or rounding through the back, hinge at the hips by pushing your glutes backward. Picture "closing a door with your glutes"—this visual cue helps reinforce the right movement pattern, activating the glutes as the primary movers (DeLuca, 2015).

Keep Your Knees Aligned with Your Toes

To prevent stress on your knees and ensure proper glute engagement, keep your knees aligned with your toes during squats, lunges, and step-ups. You should be able to see your toes by looking over your knees whenever you bend them to be sure you have not bent them too far. This alignment becomes even more crucial when using added resistance. Avoid letting your knees collapse inward (valgus), as this places undue strain on the knees and reduces glute activation. Maintaining this alignment improves overall stability, distributing the workload more effectively to the glutes (Biel, 2014).

Limit Knee Bend in Certain Movements

Avoid bending the knees too much or letting them extend excessively forward in exercises like hip thrusts or glute bridges. An ideal knee angle is around 90 degrees, which allows the glutes to work more effectively and reduces stress on the quads. Keeping the knees in this optimal position helps direct the focus back to the glutes and protects the knees from unnecessary strain (McGill, 2015).

Use a Controlled, Full Range of Motion

Moving through a full range of motion without rushing enhances glute activation and control. This is particularly important in the eccentric (lowering) phase, where the muscles lengthen under tension. For example, lowering your hips slowly and rising with control in hip thrusts ensures that the glutes are fully engaged. Likewise, during squats and lunges, descending until you feel the glutes activated—and pressing back up without bouncing—keeps the movement targeted and prevents momentum from taking over (DeLuca, 2015).

Engage Your Core Throughout the Movement

Core engagement is critical for stability and protecting the spine from unnecessary stress. Bracing your core during squats, lunges, and deadlifts helps keep the pelvis stable and prevents the lower back from arching. A helpful cue is to imagine pulling your navel toward your spine, reinforcing core stability and allowing you to maintain better posture during each lift (Contreras & Schoenfeld, 2011).

Keep Your Feet Positioned Correctly

Foot positioning can significantly impact which muscles are engaged. For example, positioning your feet shoulder-width apart or slightly wider can shift the emphasis onto the glutes in squats and lunges. A somewhat wider stance generally engages the glutes more, while a narrow stance can over-rely on the quads. Experiment with your foot placement to find the position that best activates your glutes while keeping the movement comfortable and balanced (Biel, 2014).

Avoid Excessive Leaning or Tilting

Excessive leaning, especially in exercises like Bulgarian split squats or lunges, can transfer the load to the lower back and compromise the glutes' engagement. To keep your torso relatively upright, try performing these exercises near a mirror to monitor your alignment. Avoiding forward lean reduces the risk of straining your back, keeping the focus on the glutes and providing more balanced support (McGill, 2015).

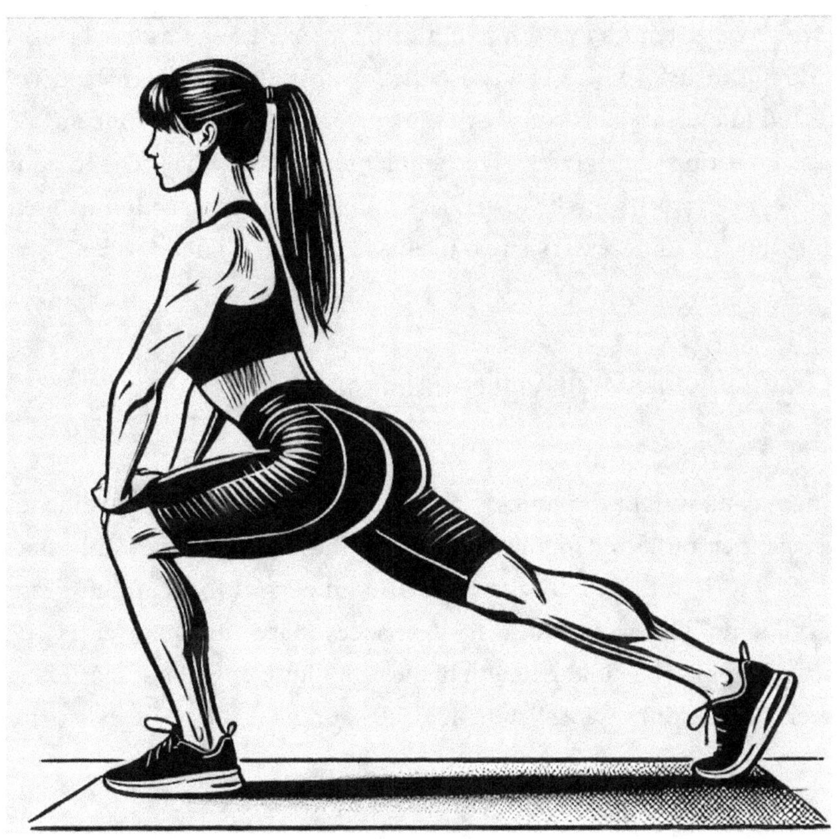

Lunge with Torso Upright

Monitor Your Pelvic Position in Glute Bridges and Hip Thrusts

Avoid overextending your hips at the top in exercises like glute bridges and hip thrusts, which can cause the lower back to arch. Instead, try a slight pelvic tuck as you reach the movement's top and concentrate on squeezing your glutes. This adjustment directs the focus to your glutes and away from the lower back, maximizing contraction without introducing unnecessary stress (DeLuca, 2015; Jetdigitaldev, 2023).

Gradually Increase Weight to Maintain Control

Increasing weight too quickly can lead to compensatory movements, with other muscles stepping in to support the load. To prevent this, start with a weight that allows you to maintain perfect form and increase gradually. This slow progression ensures that your glutes carry the load, helping you build strength in the right muscles without sacrificing technique (Contreras & Schoenfeld, 2011).

Putting Proper Form into Practice

By following these guidelines, you'll ensure that your movements are glute-dominant, controlled, and safe. The proper form allows you to isolate the glutes, engage them effectively, and minimize the overuse of other muscle groups while lowering the risk of injury. Practicing these form principles consistently helps you build a strong foundation for glute strength, supporting your everyday physical activities and enhancing your training over time (McGill, 2015).

The correct form makes your workouts more effective and each movement safer, allowing you to focus on targeting the glutes without placing unnecessary strain on other muscles or joints. With these techniques, you can confidently move forward in your glute training, knowing that your form is intentional and precise. As you progress, remember that control and technique are the foundation of any successful glute-focused workout program (DeLuca, 2015).

6

Chapter 6

Progressive Overload

Building stronger, more resilient glutes isn't about just going through the motions; it requires a deliberate approach to gradually increase the challenge on your muscles. This concept, progressive overload, is a core principle in strength training. It involves increasing the stress on your muscles over time, prompting them to adapt and grow stronger. When it comes to glute training, applying progressive overload helps you continuously challenge your glutes and avoid plateaus, ensuring that you're maximizing each workout (DeLuca, 2015). This chapter explores ways to incorporate progressive overload into your glute workouts so you can keep seeing progress as you get stronger.

Ways to Implement Progressive Overload

Gradually Increase Weight or Resistance

One of the most effective progressive overload methods is gradually increasing the weight you're lifting. You continuously challenge your glutes without sacrificing form by adding small increments to exercises like hip thrusts, squats, or deadlifts. Start with a weight that allows you to perform each rep with reasonable control, then add 5-10 pounds over time as you feel stronger. For example, if you're performing hip thrusts with a barbell, consider adding a small amount of weight each week or every other week, depending on your progress and comfort (Contreras & Schoenfeld, 2011).

Add Resistance Bands

Resistance bands are a versatile tool that can enhance glute activation, especially in movements like glute bridges, squats, or hip abductions. Placing a resistance band around your thighs or knees adds extra tension, keeping your glutes engaged throughout the movement, particularly at the peak of contraction. Begin with a light band and gradually work up to a heavier one as your glutes become stronger (Biel, 2014; Corefx, 2023; Lyfta, 2023).

Increase Reps or Sets

Increasing the number of repetitions or sets in your workout adds to the total workload, promoting muscle endurance and growth. Gradually raise the number of reps or sets while maintaining good form. For instance, if you're doing Bulgarian split squats with 3 sets of 8 reps, try moving up to 3 sets of 10 reps, then eventually to 4 sets. This incremental increase in workload keeps your muscles working harder each time (McGill, 2016; Research, 2024; Coburn & Coburn, 2022).

Slow Down the Tempo

Controlling the tempo of each rep, particularly the eccentric (lowering) phase, increases the time under tension, which makes each movement more challenging. Try slowing down the lowering phase to about 3-4 seconds, engaging the glutes more intentionally. For example, when performing hip thrusts, lower your hips over three seconds, then rise back up with control, squeezing the glutes at the top (Contreras & Schoenfeld, 2011).

Increase Range of Motion (ROM)

Expanding the range of motion in your exercises can add an extra stretch to your glutes, activating them more effectively. For example, you can modify some exercises, such as performing deficit reverse lunges or deeper squats, to engage your glutes through a broader range. However, if you experience knee pain when doing this, you have bent your knees too far. For lunges, try placing your front foot on a small step or platform to increase the depth of the movement, adding more stretch and activation to the glutes (DeLuca, 2015).

Use Single-Leg Variations for Added Challenge

Single-leg exercises can significantly increase the intensity of glute-focused movements by isolating each glute individually. Exercises like single-leg hip thrusts, single-leg Romanian deadlifts, or Bulgarian split squats emphasize each glute, requiring more stabilization and focus. As you progress, try transitioning from two-leg to single-leg versions of specific exercises, like moving from a standard hip thrust to a single-leg hip thrust, to increase the workload on each glute (McGill, 2015).

Increase the Frequency of Glute Workouts

Adding an extra glute-focused weekly workout can increase total volume, promoting muscle growth and strength. Training your glutes two to three times per week with at least a day of rest in between for recovery can be effective for progression. If you usually train your glutes once a week, consider splitting it into two shorter sessions, targeting different movements in each session (Biel, 2014).

Incorporate Heavier Compound Lifts

Compound exercises like squats and deadlifts are excellent for building glute strength. They engage multiple muscle groups while focusing significant tension on the glutes. Gradually increasing the weight while performing these compound movements is an effective way to build lower body strength. Track your progress in deadlifts and squats to ensure your glutes bear the load over time (DeLuca, 2015; Hard To Kill Fitness, 2022).

Reduce Rest Time Between Sets

Shortening your rest periods can intensify your workout, making the glutes work harder with less recovery time. Start by reducing your usual rest time by 10-15 seconds as you progress. For example, if you typically rest for 1.5 minutes between hip thrust sets, try cutting it down to 1 minute as your strength and endurance improve (Contreras & Schoenfeld, 2011).

Experiment with Drop Sets

A drop set involves performing an exercise until you're near failure, then immediately reducing the weight and continuing for more reps. This technique challenges your glutes beyond their usual capacity, ensuring they're fully engaged. To apply this in a cable kickback, for instance, perform your set with a challenging weight, then reduce the weight by 20-30% and continue for additional reps without rest, focusing on keeping the glutes engaged (McGill, 2016; 4 WAYS TO INCREASE THE INTENSITY OF YOUR WORKOUTS, n.d.).

Applying Progressive Overload Consistently

Progressive overload is not just a single technique but a long-term approach to training that keeps your muscles constantly adapting. Applying these methods gradually over time ensures that you're progressively challenging your glutes, stimulating growth, and developing strength effectively. Consistency is critical: track your progress to steadily build on each achievement, adjusting your workouts as your glutes become stronger. Whether increasing weight, changing exercises, or intensifying your tempo, small, consistent changes will lead to significant results (DeLuca, 2015).

7

Chapter 7

Glute Strength in Everyday Activities

O nce you've built strength in your glutes, the next step is learning how to incorporate that strength into your daily activities. Strong glutes provide more than just power in the gym—they also support everyday movement, stability, and ease. The fundamental transformation happened when I began consciously activating my glutes during daily tasks like bending, lifting, and walking. Reminding myself to use my glutes helped me make these tasks easier and reinforced the mind-muscle connection I had worked hard to build (Biel, 2014). One of the simplest activities to engage my glutes was stair climbing, where I could feel my glutes powering each step. This chapter will explore practical ways to activate your glutes throughout the day and in combination exercises, maximizing the benefits of your hard-earned strength.

Tips for Activating Your Glutes in Everyday Activities

Learning to engage your glutes throughout your day takes a bit of intention, but with practice, it can become second nature. Here are some ways to incorporate glute activation into daily movements:

Bending and Lifting

Every time you bend down to pick something up, you have an opportunity to activate your glutes. Rather than rounding your back or relying on your quads, try to hinge at your hips, keeping your back straight and focusing on pushing through your heels. Before lifting the object, contract your glutes and imagine they're powering the movement as you stand up. This makes lifting safer for your back and trains your glutes to engage when you need extra support (McGill, 2015).

Walking

Glute activation during walking can reduce the load on your quads and minimize stress on your knees. Focus on pushing off through your heels rather than your toes with each step to activate your glutes as you walk. This makes it easier to activate your glutes while you are walking. Imagine your glutes driving your stride rather than relying solely on your legs. You may also find it helpful to squeeze your glutes lightly with each step, especially if you're walking uphill or up an incline, which naturally calls for more glute involvement (Contreras & Schoenfeld, 2011).

Stair Climbing

Stair climbing is a natural way to engage your glutes, involving hip extension and upward movement. When climbing stairs, focus on pressing through the heel of your front foot and squeezing your glutes to lift your body. Rather than pushing off with your lower leg, consider each step an opportunity to power upward with your glutes. This practice activates the glutes, helps you move more efficiently, and reduces the load on your knees (DeLuca, 2015).

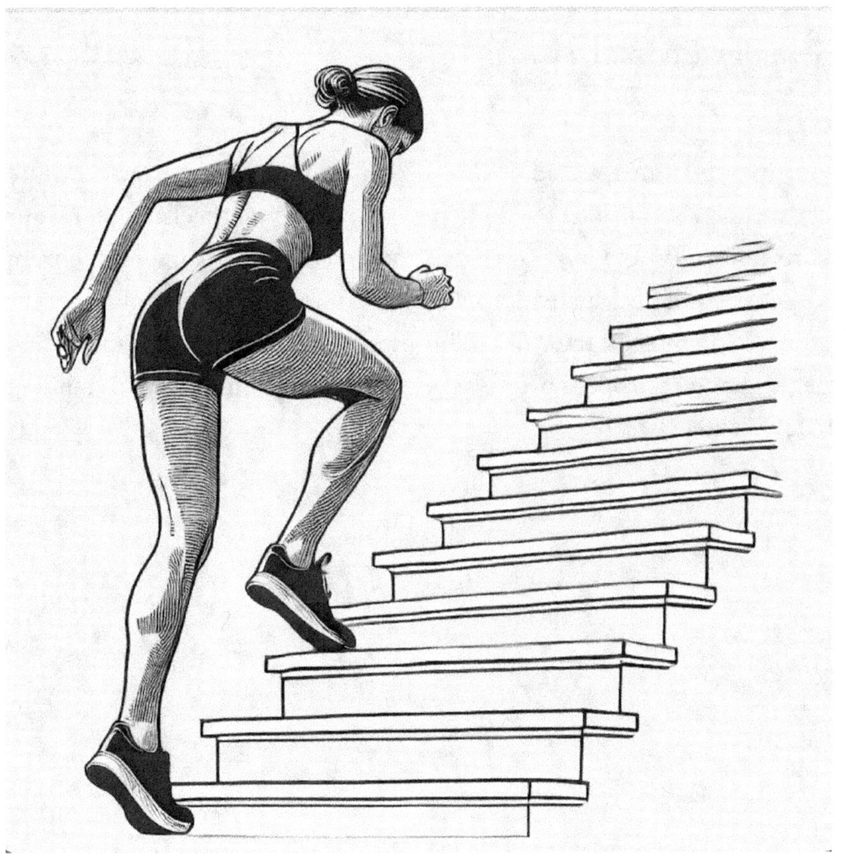

Stair Climbing

Standing Up from a Chair

Getting up from a seated position is an ideal chance to practice glute activation. As you start to stand, press through your heels, tighten your core, and contract your glutes to lift yourself. Avoid using momentum to get up quickly. Instead, focus on a controlled rise, allowing your glutes to do most of the work. This practice reinforces hip stability and helps maintain proper posture as you transition from sitting to standing (McGill, 2015).

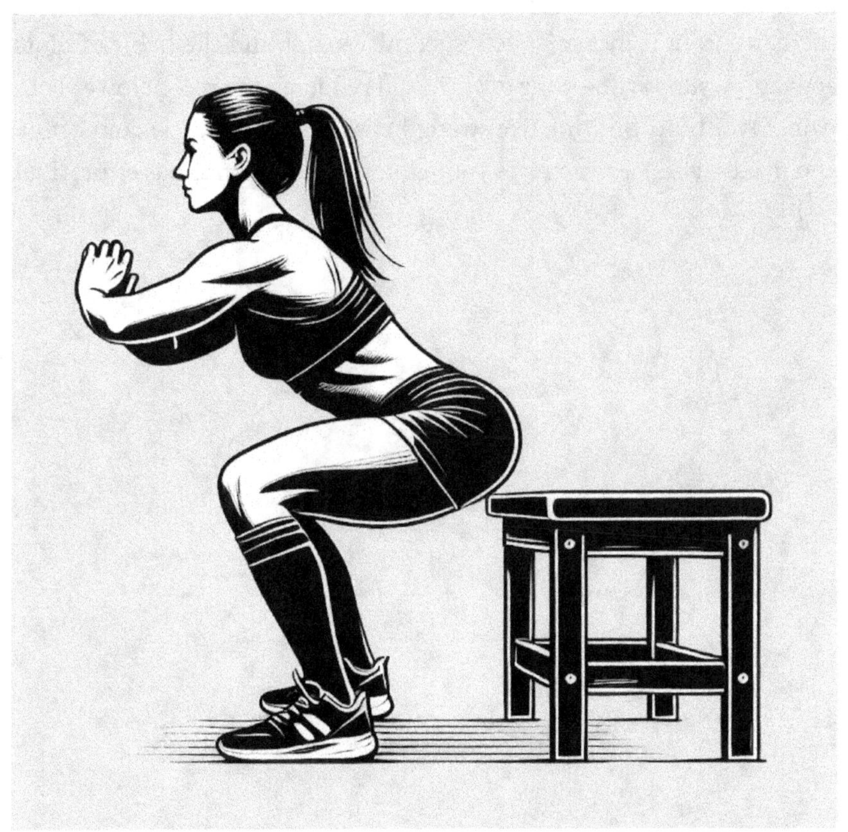

Standing Up from a Stool

Maintaining Proper Posture Throughout the Day

Good posture relies heavily on glute engagement. Try to maintain a neutral pelvis by tucking your glutes slightly and aligning your spine when standing or sitting. Regularly contracting your glutes throughout the day—even if just for a few seconds—can build the habit of glute activation, supporting your posture and reducing the risk of lower back pain. Over time, this practice strengthens the mind-muscle connection and makes it easier to activate your glutes without conscious effort (Biel, 2014).

8

Chapter 8

Using Glutes in Combination Exercises

Combination exercises engage multiple muscle groups, often including the glutes and other areas like the core, legs, or upper body. Incorporating glute activation into these exercises increases their efficiency. It strengthens your awareness of how to use your glutes as part of a full-body movement, which will enhance the incorporation of glute strength into everyday activities.

Lunges with Overhead Press

Lunges naturally activate the glutes, but adding an overhead press to this movement challenges your balance and core stability. As you lunge forward, focus on driving through your front heel and contracting your glutes to stabilize yourself. When you push back up to standing, squeeze your glutes at the top and press the weight overhead, keeping your core engaged. This combination of lower- and upper-body work makes each rep more challenging, reinforcing your glute engagement (Contreras & Schoenfeld, 2011).

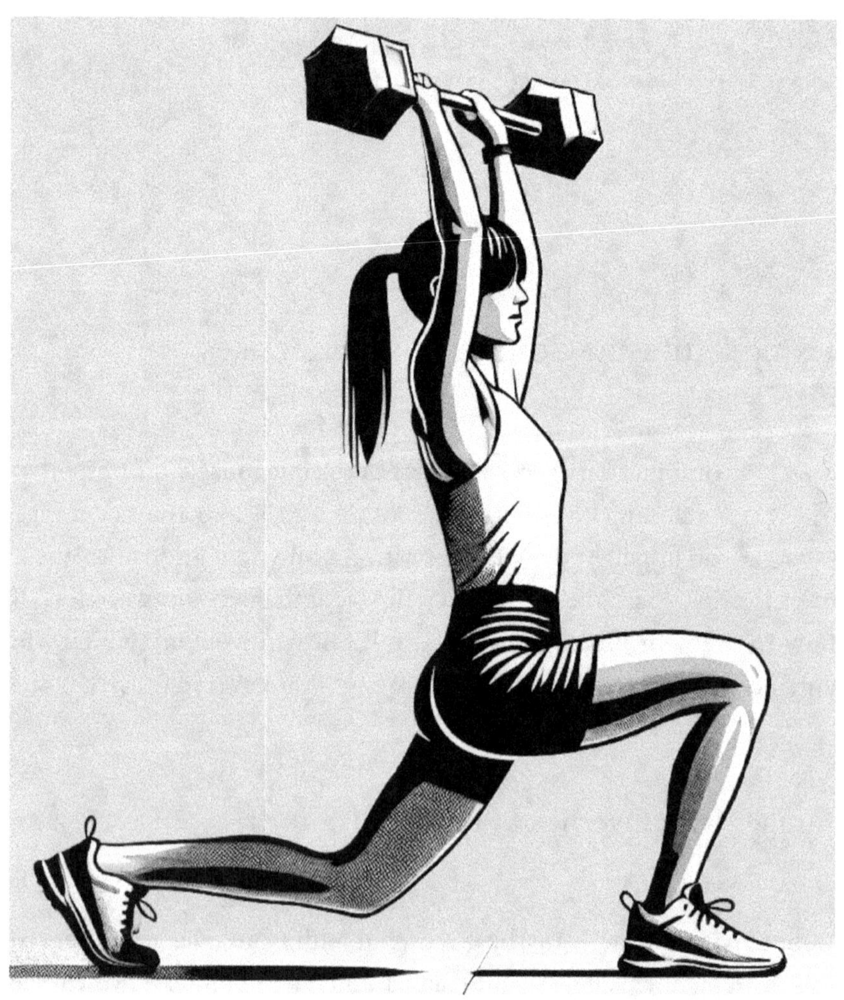

Lunge with Overhead Press

Deadlifts with Row

Deadlifts are excellent for glute activation, and combining them with a row further engages your upper back and core. Start by performing a hip hinge, focusing on pushing your glutes back and keeping your spine neutral. As you lift back up, squeeze your glutes and perform a row at the top of the movement. Focusing on glute activation during the hinge and return effectively combines lower-body and upper-body strength (McGill, 2015).

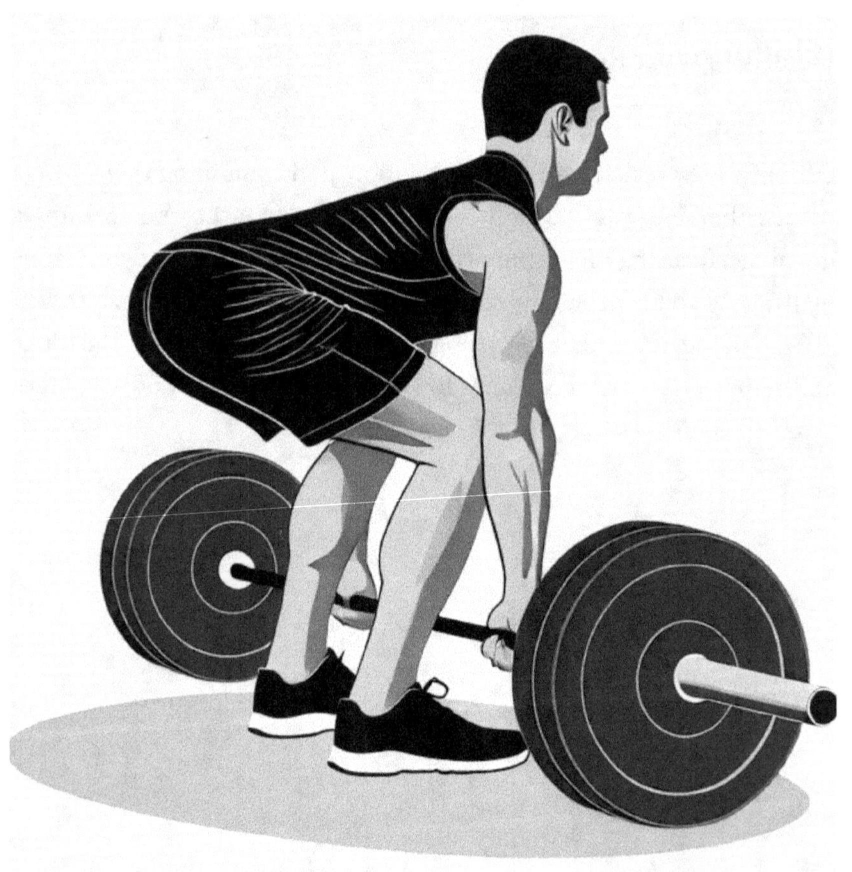

Deadlift Start with Hip Hinge, Glutes Back, and Neutral Spine

Squat to Shoulder Press

Adding an overhead press to your squat requires glute engagement and helps maintain stability as you lift the weight. Perform a standard squat, pressing through your heels to activate your glutes as you rise, then immediately press the weight overhead. Focus on engaging your glutes and core to keep the movement steady and controlled. This combination reinforces the habit of activating your glutes every time you squat (DeLuca, 2015).

Step-Up to Knee Raise

This movement combines a step-up with a knee raise, which requires balance and core engagement. Step onto a box or bench, pressing through your heel and activating your glute to lift yourself. At the top, raise your opposite knee, which forces your standing leg's glute to stabilize you. Focus on maintaining balance and a strong glute contraction as you raise your knee. This combination exercise is excellent for glute activation and stability (Biel, 2014).

Bulgarian Split Squat with Bicep Curl

Bulgarian split squats are naturally glute-focused, and adding a bicep curl to the movement also engages the upper body. As you lower into the squat, concentrate on driving through the heel of your front foot, squeezing your glute as you push back up. At the top, perform a bicep curl, keeping your core steady and maintaining control. This exercise challenges your balance and glute activation while involving the arms (Contreras & Schoenfeld, 2011).

Making Glute Activation a Habit

Activating your glutes throughout your day and during combination exercises helps build strength and endurance, training your body to rely on these muscles rather than overusing other areas. These practical techniques for daily activities and combined movements will make glute engagement feel more natural and intuitive over time. Eventually, you won't have to consciously remind yourself to activate your glutes—they'll automatically take on the role of stabilizing and powering your movements, reducing strain on other muscles and enhancing your physical efficiency.

Practice these strategies consistently, and glute activation will become a habit, supporting your posture, balance, and overall strength in every movement you make (McGill, 2015).

9

Conclusion

In this book, we explored the importance of strong glutes, breaking down what they are, why they matter, and how strengthening them benefits the whole body. We discussed why these exercises are considered easy—they're adaptable, accessible, and designed for gradual progress, which makes them effective yet manageable for any fitness level. This adaptability allows you to start at your own pace and progress gradually (Biel, 2014).

Starting with isolation exercises, we focused on critical movements like hip thrusts, glute bridges, and Bulgarian split squats, which specifically target the glutes while minimizing strain on other areas like the quads and lower back. We emphasized techniques for proper form, including maintaining a neutral spine, hip hinging, and keeping the knees aligned with the toes. These foundational techniques are essential for preventing the overuse of other muscles, ensuring that the glutes are the primary focus, and promoting stability throughout each exercise (DeLuca, 2015).

57

The concept of the mind-muscle connection was another focal point, with tips on slowing down movements, pausing at peak contractions, and visualizing the glutes working—all ways to ensure full glute engagement (Contreras & Schoenfeld, 2011). We also introduced the principle of progressive overload, a gradual increase in resistance that challenges the glutes to adapt and grow stronger over time. We can keep the glutes engaged and continuously improving by adding weight, adjusting reps, or incorporating resistance bands (McGill, 2016; Pyke, 2023).

We delved into the intricate glute anatomy, understanding how each part—the gluteus maximus, medius, and minimus—plays a unique role in stability, posture, and lower-body strength. This knowledge empowers you, enhancing your understanding of how to strengthen all three for improved balance, alignment, and efficient movement (Biel, 2014). Additionally, we explored how to activate the glutes in everyday activities, such as climbing stairs, lifting, and walking, as well as in combination exercises that incorporate the glutes with other muscle groups, making your glute strength functional and accessible in any setting (DeLuca, 2015).

Thank you for choosing this book to support your fitness journey. If it has been helpful, a review on Amazon would be much appreciated, as your feedback helps guide other readers and inspires me in future projects. I hope these techniques serve as a foundation for a stronger, more confident you, in both workouts and daily life.

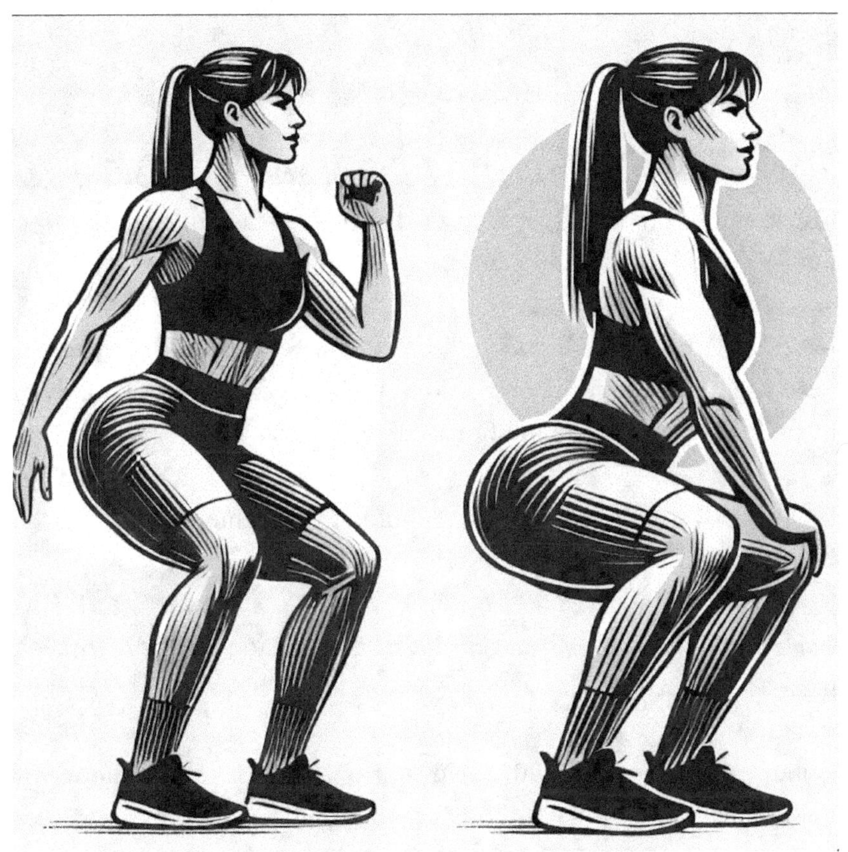

A Stronger, More Confident You

References

4 WAYS TO INCREASE THE INTENSITY OF YOUR WORKOUTS. (n.d.). https://muscleandfitnesshers.co.za/4-ways-increase-intensity-workouts/

Better active your glutes by doing THIS. (2024, November 9). [Video]. El Paso Manual Physical Therapy. Retrieved November 10, 2024, from https://www.youtube.com/shorts/8i1d5Y3hZh4

Biel, A. (2014, November 1). Trail guide to movement: Building the body in motion. *Books of Discovery.*

Cable Kickback Diagram [Image]. (2024). Shutterstock. https://www.shutterstock.com

Coburn, I., & Coburn, I. (2022, November 1). 7 Best arm workouts for Volleyball players | Volleyball Advice. *Volleyball Advice.* https://www.volleyballadvice.com/arm-workouts-for-volleyball/#google_vignette

Coach, G. D. N. (2022, November 25). The importance of glute strength. *Body By Davis.* https://www.bodybydavis.com/post/the-importance-of-glute-strength

Collins, K. (2019, April 8). *7 Butt Exercises You Can Do with Bad Knees - No Squats Needed.* Paleo Blog. https://blog.paleohacks.com/butt-exercises-can-do-with-bad-knees/

Contreras, B., & Schoenfeld, B. (2011). To crunch or not to crunch: An Evidence-Based Examination of spinal flexion exercises, their potential risks, and their applicability to program design. *Strength and Conditioning Journal*, 33(4), 8–18. https://doi.org/10.1519/ssc.0b013e3 182259d05

Corefx. (2023, May 31). *Workouts*. https://corefx.ca/blogs/workouts

DeLuca, T. (2015). NSCA's guide to program design. Human Kinetics.

Fitness, M. (2023, June 8). *Hex Bar Deadlift: Tips and techniques for form and safety*. MAGMA Fitness. https://magmafitness.com/blogs/magma-blog/hex-bar-deadlift-tips-and-techniques-for-form-and-safety?shpxi d=4aa7a729-c507-48b6-9bdd-e39782068e1b

Hard To Kill Fitness. (2022, January 20). Exercises to help you run faster and build power. *Hard To Kill Fitness*. https://hardtokillfitness.co/blogs /fitness-articles/exercises-to-help-you-run-faster-and-build-power

In silico methods to evaluate Fracture Risk and Bone Mineral Density changes in patients undergoing Total Hip Replacement - AMS Tesi di Laurea - AlmaDL - Università di Bologna. (n.d.). https://amslaurea.unibo.it/1 1058/

Jetdigitaldev. (2023, August 31). *5 tips for preventing hamstring Injuries | Genesis orthopaedic and spine*. Genesis Orthopaedic and Spine. https://g samedicine.com/5-tips-for-preventing-hamstring-injuries/

Johnson, K. S. (2023). An exploration of movement and handling by physiotherapists in a rehabilitation setting: a motion analysis study. *rgu-repository.worktribe.com*. https://doi.org/10.48526/rgu-wt-207166 7

Lyfta. (2023, November 23). *Lateral step-up video guide* [Video]. https://www.lyfta.app/exercise/lateral-step-up-6p6

McGill, S. (2015). *Low back disorders: Evidence-based Prevention and Rehabilitation.* Human Kinetics.

Menichetti, A. (2016). IN SILICO METHODS TO EVALUATE FRAC-TURE RISK AND BONE MINERAL DENSITY CHANGES IN PA-TIENTS UNDERGOING TOTAL HIP REPLACEMENT. In L. Cristo-folini, P. Gargiulo, & M. K. Gíslason, *LABORATORIO DI MECCANICA DEI TESSUTI BIOLOGICI* [Thesis]. https://core.ac.uk/download/7837 2934.pdf

Naskar, A. (2023, December 5). *8 best fabric Resistance Bands.* STYLE-CRAZE. https://www.stylecraze.com/articles/best-fabric-resistance-b ands/

OpenAI. (2024). Black and white illustrations of persons performing various exercises [AI-generated images]. DALL-E.

OpenAI. (2024). ChatGPT (Model GPT-4) [Large language model]. Retrieved October 28, 2024, from https://chat.openai.com

Personal Training | Perpetual Movement Fitness | JP Purkey | Boulder, CO. (n.d.). PMF. https://www.perpetualmovementfitness.com/cake2

Pt, B. D. B. M. (2023, August 3). 5 Must-Try Leg Press Exercises to target and tone your glutes. *Exercise With Style.* https://exercisewithsty le.com/leg-press-for-glutes/

Pyke, E. (2023, July 10). *How to Get Toned Glutes with a Rowing Machine.*

Fit Shape. https://www.fitshape.com.au/cardio/rowing-machine/glutes-workout/

Rachelle. (2024, February 26). How to prevent shoulder injuries? | Healthstin. *Just For The Health Of It! - HEALTHSTIN.* https://www.healthstin.com.au/how-can-we-prevent-shoulder-injuries/

Research, A. I. (2024, August 7). *Knee extension: definition, how it works, best knee extension workouts and benefits - Athletic Insight.* Athletic Insight. https://www.athleticinsight.com/exercise/leg/knee-extension

Richter, D. (2023, May 19). *How many exercises should you do per muscle group? (Guide).* StrengthLog. https://www.strengthlog.com/how-many-exercises-per-muscle-group/

Rush, B. (2024, June 24). *6 Best Pregnancy Exercises for Women - Louisville Mom Collective.* Louisville Mom Collective. https://louisvillemomcollective.com/pregnancy/6-best-pregnancy-exercises/

Weak glutes are affecting your knee pain! (2024, November 2). [Video]. El Paso Manual Physical Therapy. Retrieved November 3, 2024, from https://www.youtube.com/shorts/lM1Ij_5KnxY

Woman in a Park Performing Standing Kickback with Resistance Band [Cover Photograph]. (2024). Shutterstock. https://www.shutterstock.com

Woman in a Park Performing Glute Bridge [Cover Photograph]. (2024). Shutterstock. https://www.shutterstock.com

9 798300 208790